F Is for Fluoride

A Feasible Fairytale
for Freethinkers
15 and Up

Forrest F. Freelander, F.F.D.

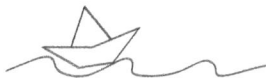

Internet addresses included in this book were accurate at the time of publishing. The information in this book is for informational purposes only and is not a substitute for medical advice from a knowledgeable healthcare provider.

ISBN 978-1-7324022-0-1

For Andy, Sue, David, Ella, Sim, and baby Roo

For Gia, Ginger, Buster, Elvis I and Elvis II

For my front lawn and potted plants

(they drink tap water, too)

For little me when I was three

and big dreamers like you

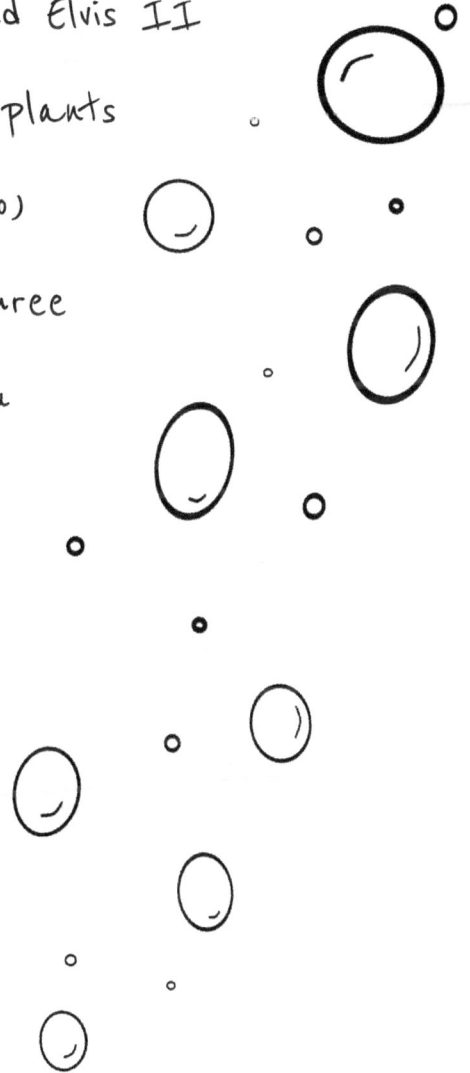

- F -

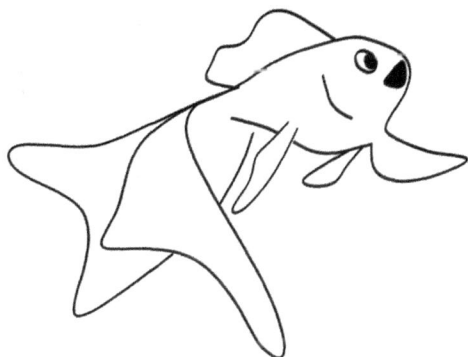

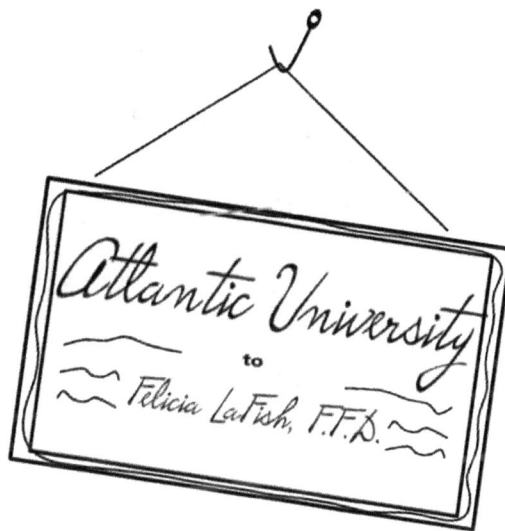

F is for fluoride, fantastic, fun, fine, fairy, fish, and finally.
How fitting this fun fairytale is finally told by a _fantastic_ fish like me!
My name is Dr. Felicia LaFish and I just happen to be
a fine dentist—therefore fluoride is my specialty.

My friends and I pump fluoride through your water pipes

all the livelong day.

We mix it in your toothpaste to keep cavities at bay.

We can even make it taste like bubble-gum

(at least that's what we say)

and we've been doing it for decades,

as if it's always been this way.

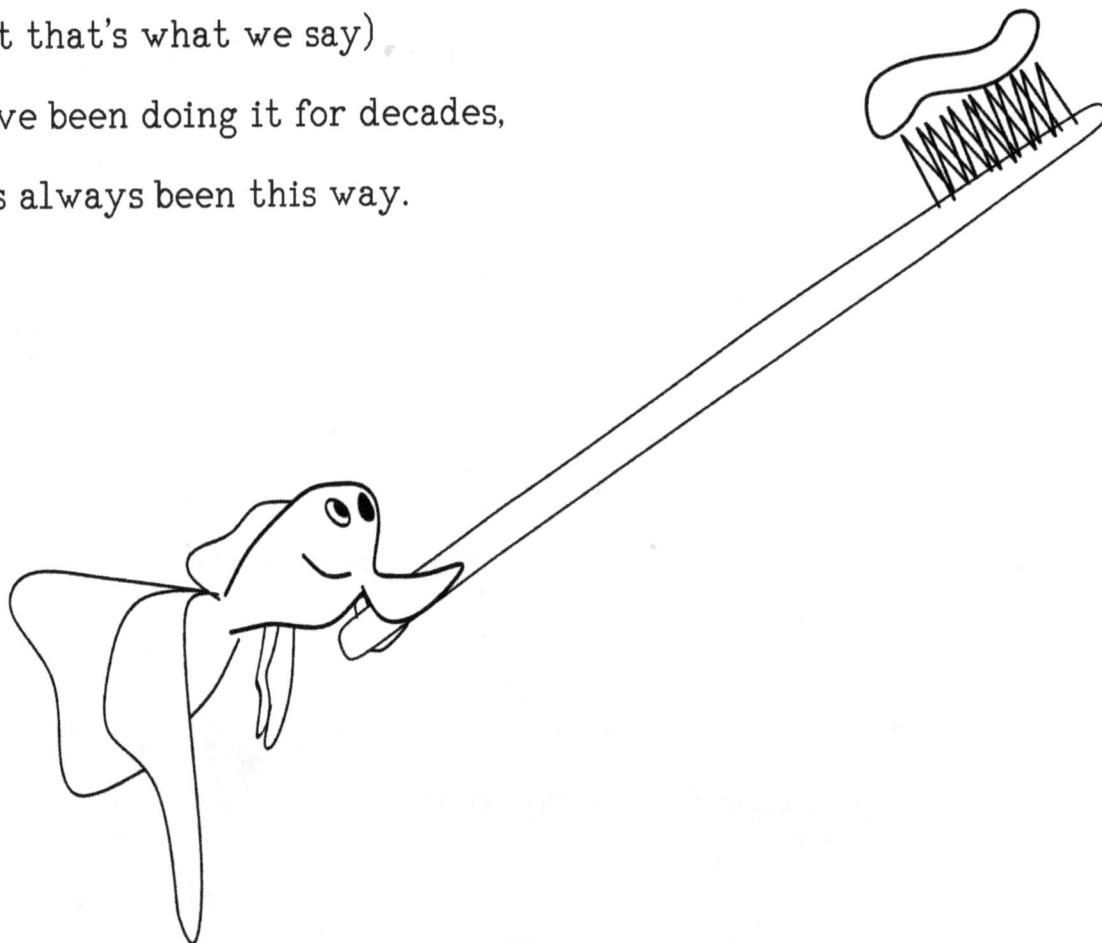

2

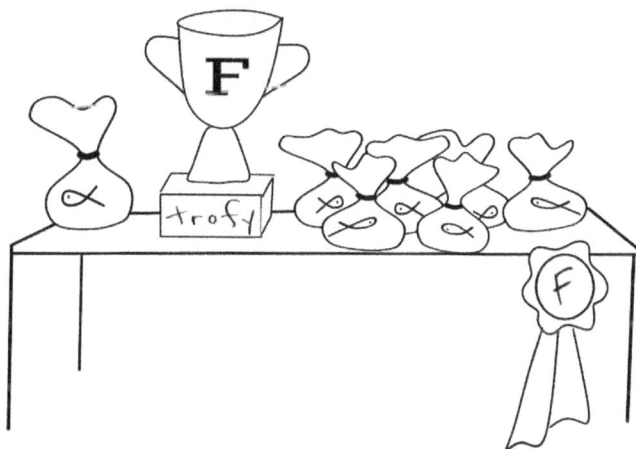

Fluoride Fair

The fruit of our effort is clear, so says the CDC.

Children with fluoride in their water have, on average, two less cavities.[1]

It's one of the greatest public health triumfs of the past century[2]

—if we do say so ourselves, that seems like quite a feat indeed.

But I noticed something recently that has me scratching my head;

the rate of cavities dropped equally where fluoridation has not spread.[3]

And something else caught my attention, just last month I read

a team of Harvard professors cautioned fluoride is a neurotoxin like lead.[4]

Drop in Rate of Cavities

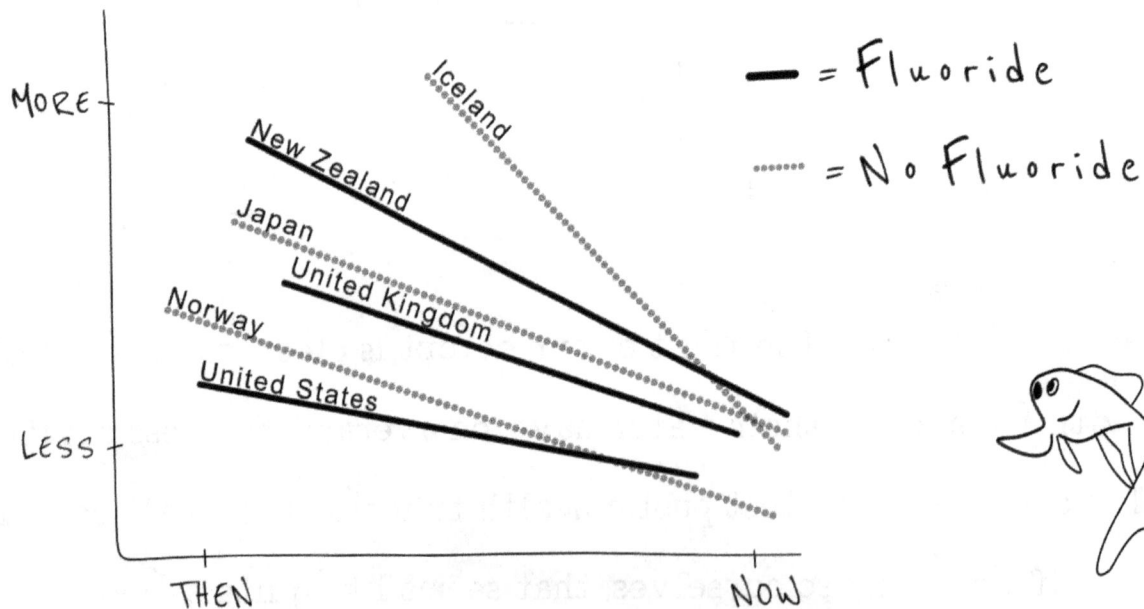

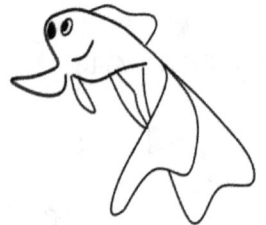

MORE

LESS

Iceland

New Zealand

Japan

United Kingdom

Norway

United States

—— = Fluoride

······· = No Fluoride

THEN   NOW

*Table F derived from data from World Health Organization, see reference 3

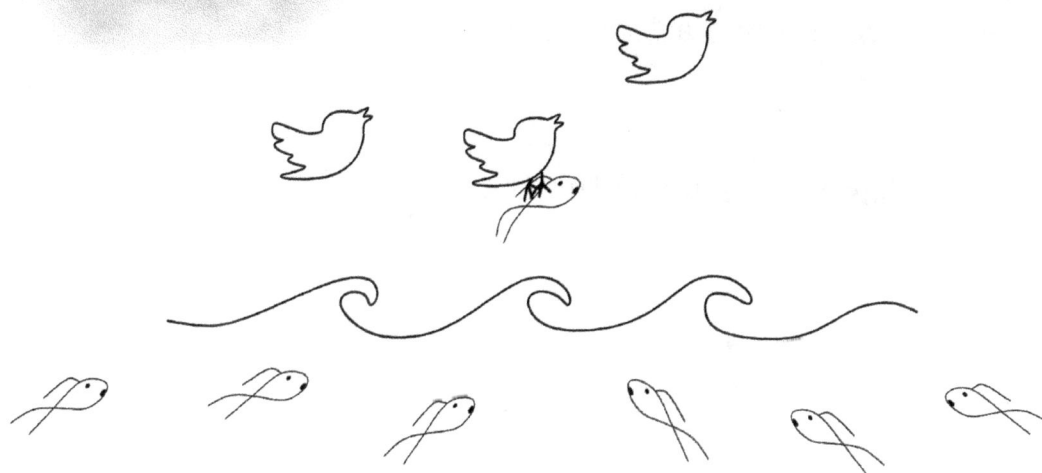

Now, I thought anti-fluoride folk were looneys on the street

but scientists say longterm studies of fluoridation are incomplete.[5]

Sweden's Nobel-winning neuropharmacologist called fluoride obsolete.[6]

Even leading dentists who once endorsed it admit there was deceit.[7]

(Just ask Dr. Hardy Limeback in Canada who now sends tweet after tweet

trying to warn you of fluoride's health effects.[8] It really is quite sweet.)

Here is where our "once upon a time" comes into play

—if fluoride's not the prince we think it is,

why do we drink it to this day?

We don't add other drugs to the water supply

or push them in this way.

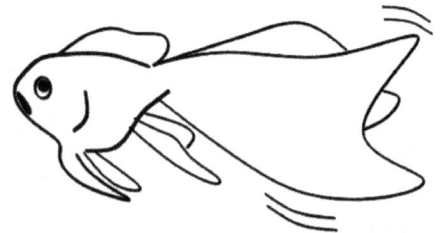

There's a reason fluoride's special,

and the price is ours to pay.

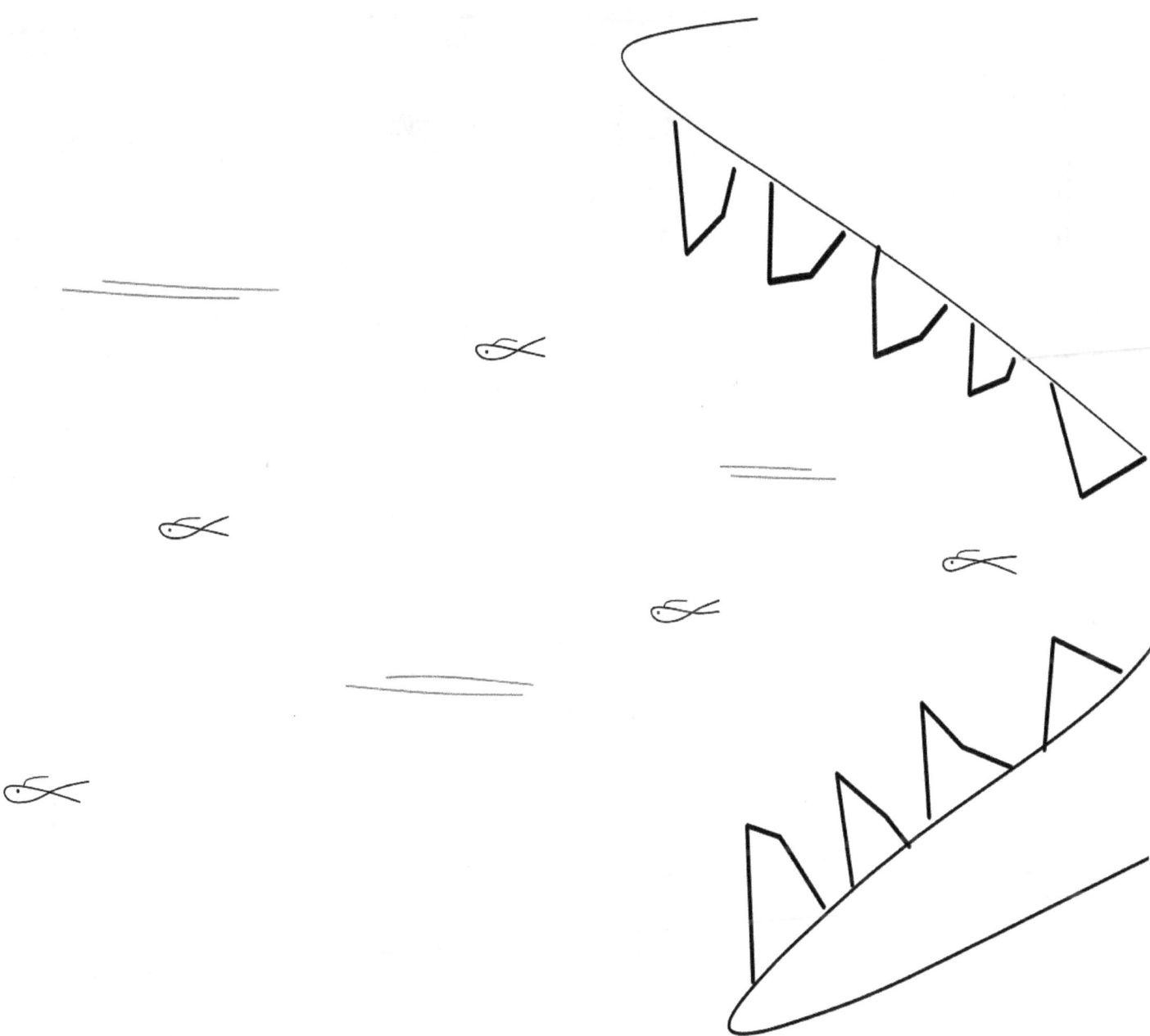

Once upon a time,

in a world weary from war,

fluoride flooded into the atmosphere

from factories galore.

It was a leading air pollutant,

leaving lawsuits in its wake,[9]

'til corporate lawyers banded together

—they knew what was at stake.

They founded institutes and research labs

and "helped" direct their work.[10]

Sure, the "science" all supported fluoride

but that was just a perk. ;)

Dentists who endorsed it

moved up and up and up

while dissenters who dissented

were kicked out of the club.

When a national dental institute was formed,

they knew just the man

to direct the new federal agency

and carry out their plan.

Thanks to his infatuation with water fluoridation,

he began the first trial three years before.[11]

Two years later the government declared fluoride

safe and effective for everyone

forevermore.

~~THE END~~

It's no surprise fluoride was approved

ten years before the first trial was through

or that the fluoride added to water

comes direct from a factory smokestack to you.[12]

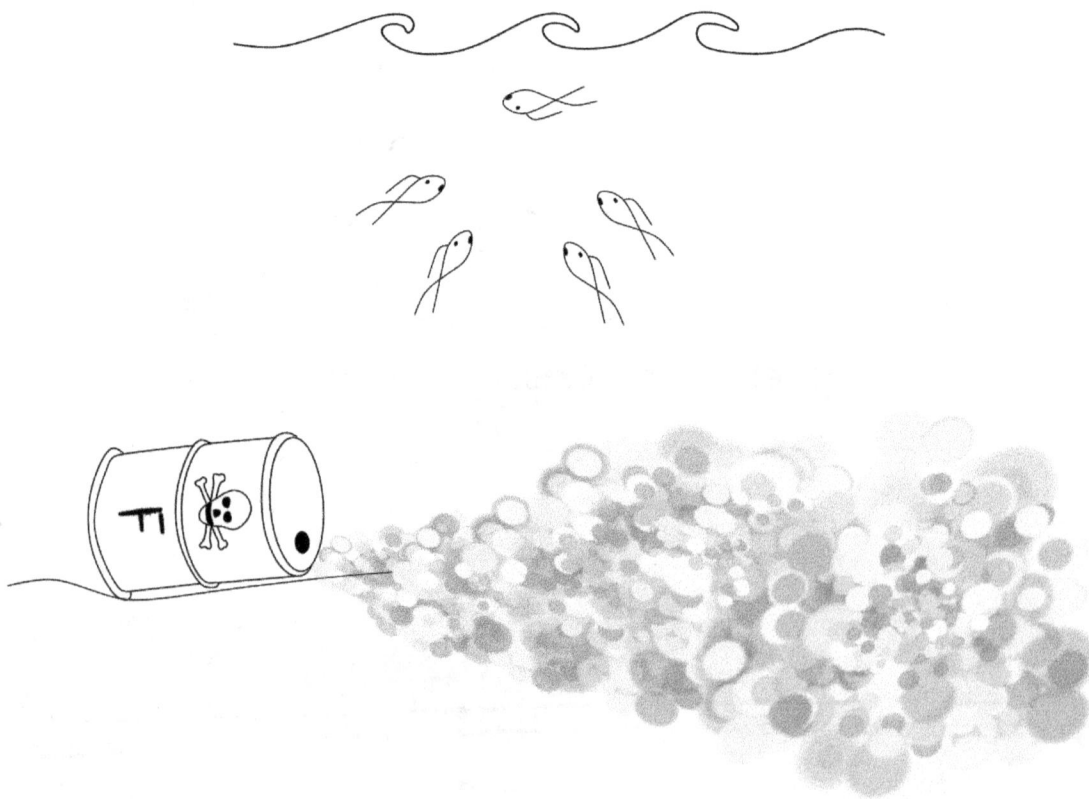

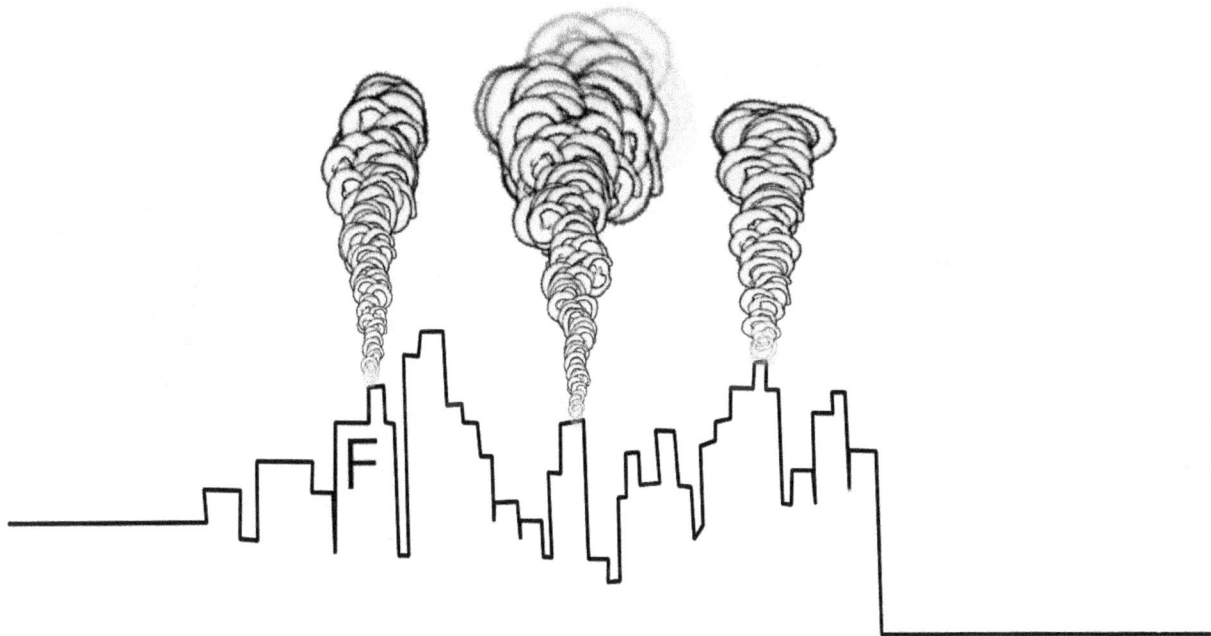

The head of the federal health department, at the time,

was fluoride-friendly, too;

he was fresh off the roster as a lawyer for the number one polluter[13]

—cliché, I know, but true.

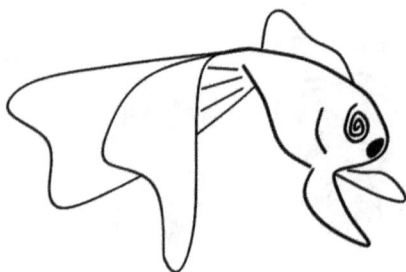

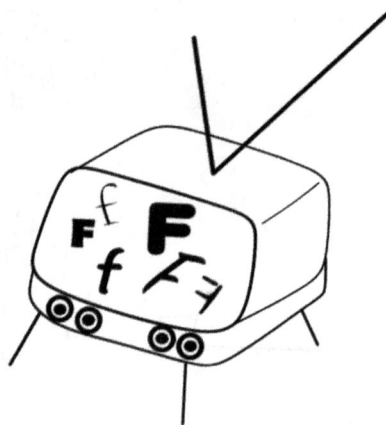

Once fluoridation was approved,

that was just the beginning.

Next, they hired a marketing magician

to keep your pretty head spinning.

Sigmund Freud was his uncle

and propaganda was his game.[14]

He's the guy who got experts to promote cigarettes,

and with fluoride he did the same.[15]

He also leveraged authority figures

like dictionaries and the daily news

to foster the fallacy that fluoride is safe and effective,

and snuff out opposing views.

12

Maybe we fell for these tricks back then, you say,

but our modern minds are more savvy?

After all, dumping toxic waste in the water to treat children

does sound a little psychopath-y.

Surely our current experts would have exposed

such a scheme so long in the making

—except dentistry is dictated by sugar execs now

who don't really care about teeth.[16]

(they're just faking)

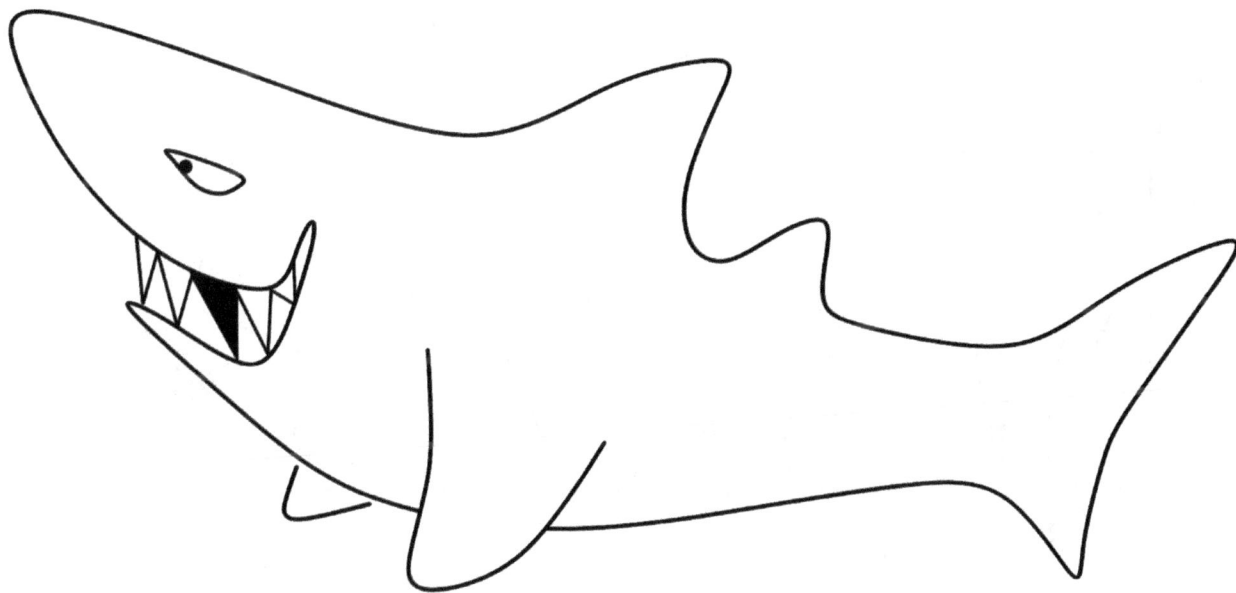

Dentists will tell you fluoride is natural in some water sources

and this fact, I affirm, is true

but just because something is found naturally in nature

does not mean it is good for you.

Freshwater is typically very low in fluoride,

much lower than what dentists suggest,[17]

and countless studies reveal a dark side to fluoridation

but their findings have been suppressed.

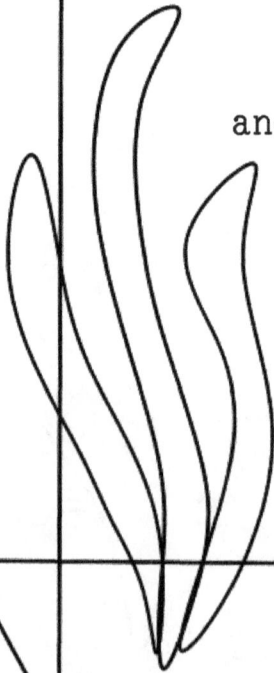

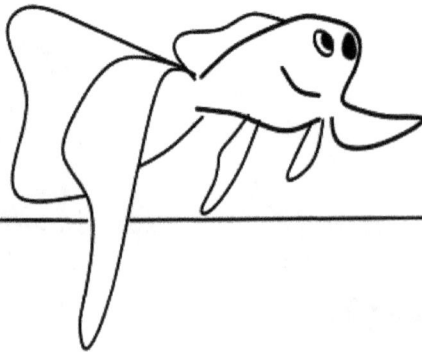

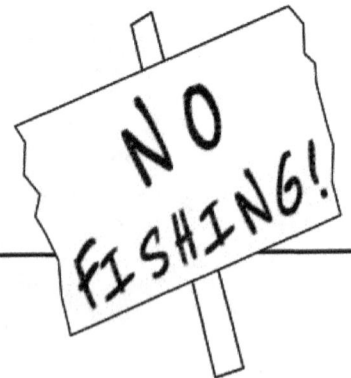

NO FISHING!

It's long been known fluoride accumulates in bone,

causing symptoms of arthritis.[18]

It also depresses the thyroid,

like Hashimoto's thyroiditis.[19]

It calcifies heavily in the pineal gland,[20]

a brain organ that regulates sleep.

Even dentists admit it discolors tooth enamel[21]

—lucky for them, to fix it isn't cheap.

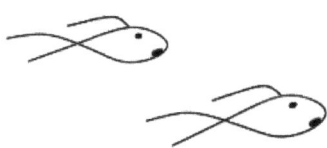

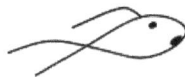

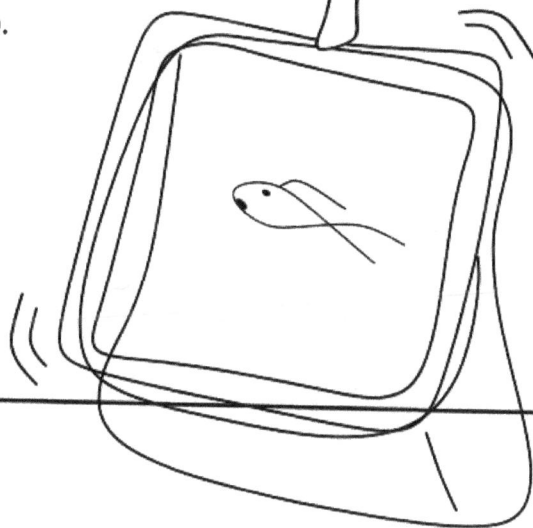

But the scariest part of fluoride's health effects

is what doctors don't yet know.

Studies of pregnancy and the elderly

should've been done decades ago.[22]

It took an FBI intelligence analyst

to point out fluoride causes acne.[23]

That book should have been written, critics claim,

by a medical doctor, or at least a PhD.

Exactly.

Experts who question fluoride are ostracized

—or worse.

To tackle the dental darling

is to afflict your career

with a fated curse.[24]

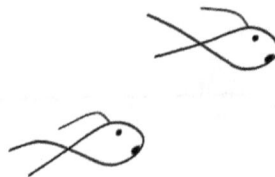

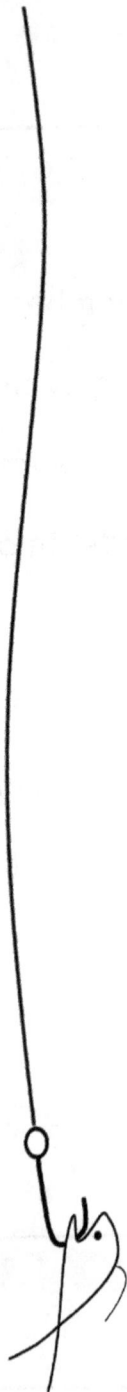

William Marcus was fired from the EPA

when a study linked fluoride with cancer.[25]

He was reinstated under the Whistleblower Protection Act

but his concerns went unanswered.[26]

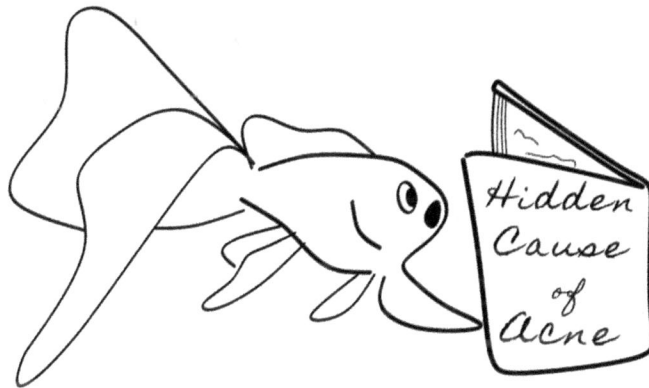

Toxicologist Phyllis Mullenix lost her funding,

and soon after, her job

when her research showed fluoride affects the function of the brain[27]

—it practically prompted a mob.[28]

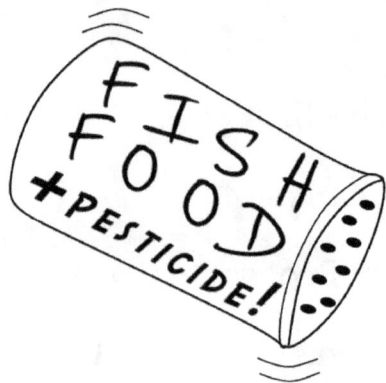

You might be thinking,

"But Felicia, isn't fluoride a nutrient found in food?"[29]

Most dentists don't know this

but the main source of fluoride in our food supply is quite crude.

You see, fluoride is a pesticide

and no one monitors its use.[30]

They figure, we dump it in the water supply,

what harm could a little more do?[31]

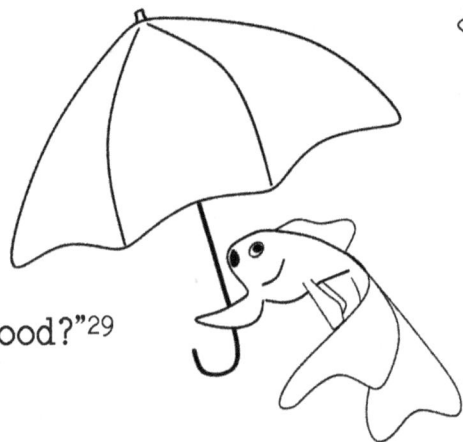

18

I'm afraid the damage done is more than anybody knows.

Poultry products are the worst because,

like us, it accumulates in their bones.[32]

And please don't get me started on fluoride

in wine, grape juice, and raisins.[33]

To be on the safe side,

here's what I advise:

stick to craisins.

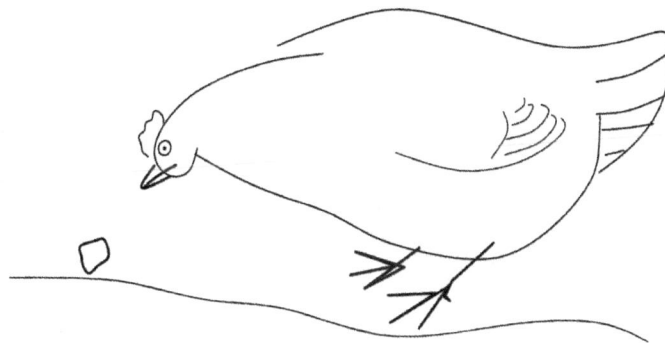

We've reached the end of our story
but our fairytale ending is still up to you.
Here are a few simple things you can do
to make all our wishes come true.

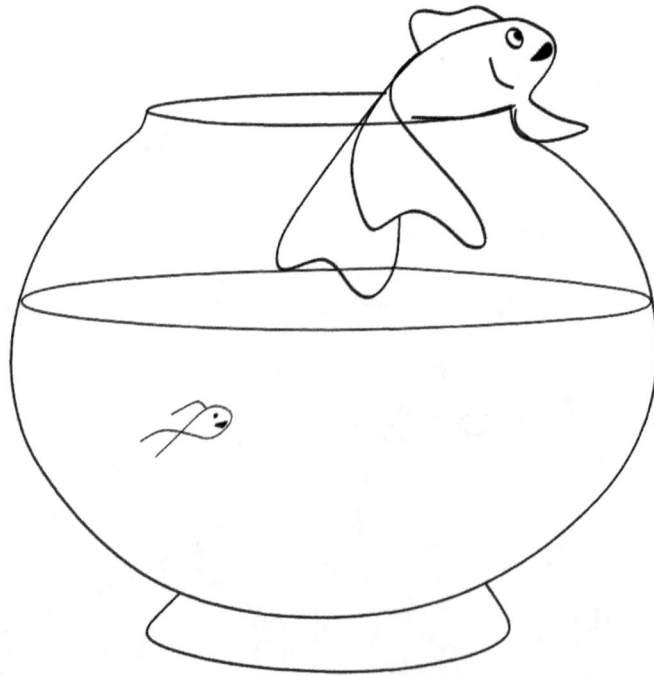

To-Do

1. Call your local politicians and tell them you want fluoride out

2. Then sign my petition demanding Congress end it now*

3. Pass this book along so before long everyone will know:

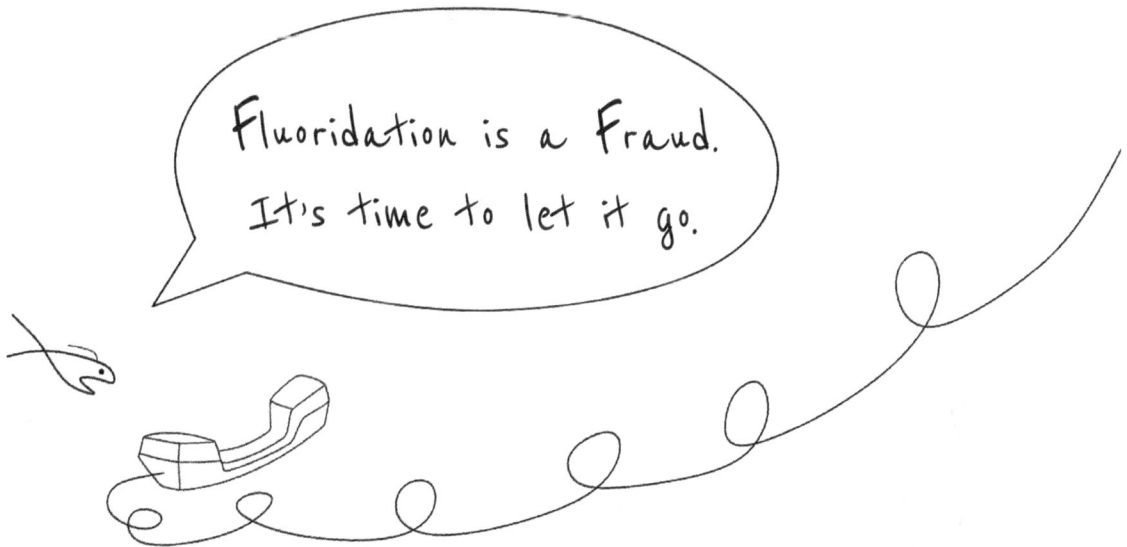

Fluoridation is a Fraud. It's time to let it go.

*To sign the petition, visit:

www.petition.projectfree.me

F is for fluoride, friendship, fitting, fearless, and finally.

How fitting fluoridation will finally end

thanks to fearless friends

like you and me.

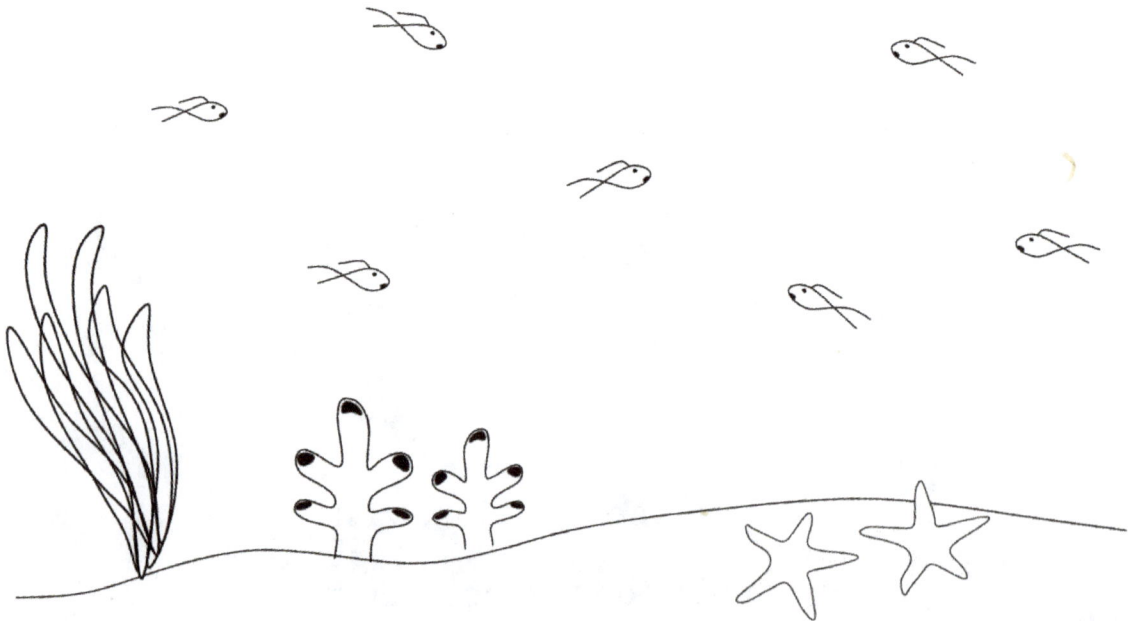

FIN

References

1. According to the CDC website, "In communities with water fluoridation, school children have, on average, about 2 fewer decayed teeth compared to children who don't live in fluoridated communities." This claim is disputed by critics of fluoridation, in part because of data from the World Health Organization that shows the rate of cavities dropped equally in countries where the water supply is not fluoridated (see reference 3 for more information). SOURCE: U.S. Centers for Disease Control and Prevention (CDC), Division of Oral Health, National Center for Chronic Disease Prevention and Health Promotion, *Over 70 Years of Community Water Fluoridation*, last modified May 14, 2017, https://www.cdc.gov/fluoridation/basics/70-years.htm.

2. The CDC named its water fluoridation program one of the top ten public health achievements of the century. SOURCE: U.S. Centers for Disease Control and Prevention (CDC), Division of Oral Health, National Center for Chronic Disease Prevention and Health Promotion, *Achievements in Public Health, 1900-1999: Fluoridation of Drinking Water to Prevent Dental Caries*, Morbidity and Mortality Weekly Report 48, no. 41 (October 22, 1999), 933-40, https://www.cdc.gov/mmwr/preview/mmwrhtml/mm4841a1.htm.

3. The chart on this page is based on data from the World Health Organization's (WHO) Collaborating Centre for Education, Training and Research in Oral Health, *Oral Health Country/Area Profile Project*, Malmö University, Sweden, http://mah.se/CAPP. See also Nicole Davis, "Is Fluoridated Drinking Water Safe?" *Harvard Public Health Magazine*, Spring 2016, https://www.hsph.harvard.edu/magazine/magazine_article/fluoridated-drinking-water/ and Douglas Main, "Fluoridation May Not Prevent Cavities, Scientific Review Shows," *Newsweek*, June 29, 2015, http://www.newsweek.com/fluoridation-may-not-prevent-cavities-huge-study-shows-348251.

4. A study published by Harvard researchers in 2012 in *Environmental Health Perspectives* concludes, "The results support the possibility of an adverse effect of high fluoride exposure on children's neurodevelopment. Future research should include detailed individual-level information on prenatal exposure, neurobehavioral performance, and covariates for adjustment." SOURCE: Ann L. Choi, Guifan Sun, Ying Zhang, and Philippe Grandjean, "Developmental Fluoride Neurotoxicity: A Systematic Review and Meta-Analysis," *Environmental Health Perspectives* 120, no. 10 (2012): 1362-68, http://nrs.harvard.edu/urn-3:HUL.InstRepos:10579664. Learn more at www.Harvard.ProjectFree.Me.

5. According to a 2015 report from the National Toxicology Program, "The existing literature is limited in its ability to evaluate potential neurocognitive effects of fluoride in people associated with the current U.S. Public Health Service drinking water guidance (0.7 mg/L)." SOURCE: U.S. Department of Health and Human Services, Division of the National Toxicology Program, *Proposed NTP Evaluation on Fluoride Exposure and Potential for Developmental Neurobehavioral Effects*, November 19, 2015, https://ntp.niehs.nih.gov/ntp/about_ntp/bsc/2015/december/meetingmaterial/fluoride_508.pdf, available at www.NTP.ProjectFree.Me.

6. "[Fluoridation] is against all principles of modern pharmacology. It's really obsolete... I think those nations that are using it should feel ashamed of themselves. It's against science." SOURCE: Arvid Carlsson, "Water Fluoridation Obsolete According to Nobel Prize Scientist," interview by Michael Connett and Chris Neurath, Fluoride Action Network, October 4, 2005, http://fluoridealert.org/content/carlsson-interview.

7. John Colquhoun was chairman of New Zealand's Fluoridation Promotion Committee and the principle dental officer of Auckland, the country's largest city. In his essay

on why he changed his mind about public water fluoridation, he reveals that he was instructed not to share mounting evidence that fluoridation is ineffective at preventing cavities. He writes, "I now realize that what my colleagues and I were doing was what the history of science shows all professionals do when their pet theory is confronted by disconcerting new evidence: they bend over backwards to explain away the new evidence. They try very hard to keep their theory intact—especially so if their own professional reputations depend on maintaining that theory." SOURCE: John Colquhoun, "Why I Changed My Mind about Fluoridation," *Perspectives in Biology and Medicine* 41, no. 1 (1997): 29-44, http://fluoridealert.org/articles/colquhoun/.

8. Hardy Limeback, D.D.S., Ph.D., is the former head of preventive dentistry at the University of Toronto and past president of the Canadian Association for Dental Research. He is also coauthor of the National Research Council's 2006 report *Fluoride in Drinking Water*. You can view his Twitter feed at https://twitter.com/DrLimeback.

9. "Airborne fluorides have caused more worldwide damage to domestic animals than any other air pollutant." SOURCE: U.S. Department of Agriculture, *Air Pollutants Affecting the Performance of Domestic Animals*, Agricultural Handbook No. 380 (1972), https://naldc.nal.usda.gov/naldc/download.xhtml?id=CAT72349227&content=PDF.

10. Fluoride polluters played a foundational role in establishing public water fluoridation. For example, the Aluminum Company of America (Alcoa) organized a self-described "Fluorine Lawyers Committee" with attorneys from U.S. Steel, Monsanto Chemical, and other corporations with a self-interest in proving fluoride safe and effective at preventing cavities. They met regularly in Washington, directed their own Medical Advisory Committee, and funded extensive research at the University of Cincinnati's Kettering Laboratory. By the 1930s, the majority of Kettering's research

focused on promoting fluoride. An Alcoa-funded researcher at the Mellon Institute in Pittsburgh made the first public proposal to add fluoride to the water supply. SOURCE: Christopher Bryson, *The Fluoride Deception* (New York: Seven Stories Press, 2011), available at www.Deception.ProjectFree.Me.

11. The initial fluoridation trial began in Grand Rapids, Michigan in 1945 by H. Trendley Dean. It was intended to be a 15-year study to compare the rate of cavities in Grand Rapids with that of a control city, but just five years into the trial, fluoride was added to water in the control city, as well, when fluoridation was prematurely endorsed by the federal government as a safe and effective way to prevent cavities. SOURCE: H. Trendley Dean et al., "Studies on Mass Control of Dental Caries through Fluoridation of the Public Water Supply," Public Health Report 65, no. 43 (1950): 1403-8, http://www.ncbi.nlm.nih.gov/pmc/articles/PMC1997106/?page=21.

12. As explained in a memo written in September 2000 by Thomas Reeves, the CDC's National Fluoridation Engineer at the time, "All of the fluoride chemicals used in the U.S. for water fluoridation, sodium fluoride, sodium fluorosilicate, and fluorosilicic acid, are useful byproducts of the phosphate fertilizer industry... These gases are captured by product recovery units (scrubbers) and condensed into 23% fluorosilicic acid." SOURCE: Thomas G. Reeves, U.S. Centers for Disease Control and Prevention, Division of Oral Health, National Center for Chronic Disease Prevention and Health Promotion, "The Manufacture of the Fluoride Chemicals," September 2000, available at http://www.fluoridealert.org/wp-content/uploads/reeves-2000.pdf.

13. The decision by the federal government to endorse public water fluoridation was made in 1950 under the leadership of Oscar Ewing, a longtime lawyer for Alcoa and the company's top legal liaison with the federal government prior to his selection in

1947 as head of the Federal Security Agency, now the Department of Health and Human Services. SOURCE: Bryson, *Fluoride Deception*, 126, available at www.Deception.ProjectFree.Me.

14. For an explanation of the "engineering of consent" and other notorious techniques used in Bernays' work, see Edward Bernays, *Propaganda* (New York: Routledge, 1928), available at www.Propaganda.ProjectFree.Me.

15. For an insightful interview with Edward Bernays and his work on fluoridation, see Bryson, *Fluoride Deception*, 160-67, available at www.Deception.ProjectFree.Me.

16. The sugar industry successfully lobbies for dental treatments like fluoride to deflect attention from the role of sugar in the development of cavities. For example, the National Caries Program (NCP) was established in 1971 with the goal of ending dental decay in a decade. When the NCP submitted their omnibus request for contracts—which set the precedent for the direction dental research would take for the decades ahead—the authors of the request copied verbatim or closely paraphrased 78 percent of a report the sugar industry submitted two years earlier. SOURCE: Cristin Kearns, Stanton A. Glantz, and Laura Schmidt, "Sugar Industry Influence on the Scientific Agenda of the National Institute of Dental Research's 1971 National Caries Program: A Historical Analysis of Internal Documents," *PLoS Medicine* 12, no. 3 (March 10, 2015), https://doi.org/10.1371/journal.pmed.1001798, available at www.Sugar.ProjectFree.Me.

17. The U.S. Public Health Service recommends fluoride levels in drinking water of 0.7 mg/L. The mean fluoride level of freshwater sources is 0.05 mg/L. SOURCE: Health Canada, *Inorganic Fluorides: Priority Substances List Assessment Report* (1993),

https://www.canada.ca/en/health-canada/services/environmental-workplace-health/reports-publications/environmental-contaminants/canadian-environmental-protection-act-priority-substances-list-assessment-report-inorganic-fluorides.html, available at www.Freshwater.ProjectFree.Me.

18. In addition to skeletal fluorosis, fluoride has long been known to cause other joint and bone issues similar to arthritis. For example, see H.A. Cook, "Fluoride Studies in Patient with Arthritis," *Lancet* 298, no. 7728 (October 9, 1971): 817. For a listing of more studies, see "Arthritis," Fluoride Action Network, accessed May 23, 2018, http://fluoridealert.org/issues/health/arthritis/. For information on other health ailments caused by fluoride, see Paul Connett, James Beck, and H. S. Micklem, *The Case Against Fluoride: How Hazardous Waste Ended Up in Our Drinking Water and the Bad Science and Powerful Politics that Keep It There* (White River Junction, VT: Chelsea Green Publishing, 2010), available at www.Case.ProjectFree.Me.

19. Until the 1950s, fluoride was used by doctors in Europe and South America to reduce thyroid function in patients with overactive thyroid glands. Even a dose of 2-5 mg per day, an amount similar to what Americans consume through fluoridated drinking water, was enough to lower thyroid function in their patients. SOURCE: Pierre Galletti and Gustave Joyet, "Effect of Fluorine on Thyroidal Iodine Metabolism in Hyperthyroidism," *Journal of Clinical Endocrinology and Metabolism* 18, no. 10 (October 1, 1958): 1102-10. See also, "Thyroid," Fluoride Action Network, accessed May 23, 2018, http://fluoridealert.org/issues/health/thyroid/.

20. In 1997, a doctoral candidate in the United Kingdom dissected eleven human pineal glands and discovered that calcified portions of the gland contain the highest concentrations of fluoride in the human body, up to 21,000 ppm. SOURCE: Jennifer Luke,

"The Effect of Fluoride on the Physiology of the Pineal Gland," (PhD diss., University of Surrey, 1997), available at http://fluoridealert.org/studiesPineal/luke-1997/.

21. Dental fluorosis is a type of discoloration and mottling of the tooth enamel caused by longterm ingestion of fluoride while the teeth are forming. According to data from national surveys conducted between 1986 and 2004, the rate of dental fluorosis among adolescents increased from 20 to 40 percent. SOURCE: Eugenio Beltrán-Aguilar, Laurie Barker, and Bruce A. Dye, "Prevalence and Severity of Dental Fluorosis in the United States, 1999-2004," National Center for Health Statistics (NCHS) Data Brief No. 53, November 2010, https://www.cdc.gov/nchs/products/databriefs/db53.htm.

22. There appears to be little interest in researching the effect of fluoride on the elderly, but a study of fluoride and pregnancy was recently conducted in Mexico by researchers with a grant from the National Institute of Environmental and Health Sciences. The study found an average loss of 2.5 to 3 IQ points for each 0.5 mg/L increase in prenatal fluoride exposure. The level of fluoride studied was similar to the amount recommended by health authorities in the United States. SOURCE: Morteza Bashash, Deena Thomas, Howard Hu, et al, "Prenatal Fluoride Exposure and Cognitive Outcomes in Children at 4 and 6-12 Years of Age in Mexico," *Environmental Health Perspectives* 125, no. 9 (September 2017), https://ehp.niehs.nih.gov/ehp655.

23. Melissa Gallico, *The Hidden Cause of Acne: How Toxic Water is Affecting Your Health and What You Can Do About It* (Rochester, VT: Healing Arts Press, 2018). For more information, see www.HiddenCauseofAcne.com.

24. For a detailed account from the early years of fluoridation, including how the American Medical Association came to endorse artificial water fluoridation without

adequate safety testing, see George Waldbott, *A Struggle with Titans* (New York: Carlton Press, 1965) available at www.Titans.ProjectFree.Me.

25. In 1977, Congress asked the National Toxicology Program (NTP) to study the role of fluoride in cancer. In 1988, the final report was submitted indicating a dose-dependent relationship between fluoride and liver cancer, as evidenced in animal studies. Instead of acting on the findings, the NTP downgraded the classification of the tumors to conclude there was no carcinogenic effect from fluoride. SOURCE: J. Sibbison, "USA: More about Fluoride," *Lancet* 336, no. 8717 (September 22, 1990): 737. See also, "Fluoride and Liver Cancers in NTP Bioassay," Fluoride Action Network, last updated April 2015, http://fluoridealert.org/studies/cancer04/.

26. When senior toxicologist William Marcus criticized the downgrading of the cancer tumors found in the NTP study mentioned above, he was subsequently fired from his position at EPA, a job he had held for 18 years. During the lengthy legal proceedings that followed, the court ruled Marcus was fired in retaliation for his stance on the fluoride study. The trial also revealed that officials at EPA falsified his time cards and made other false statements to provide justification for the illegal firing. SOURCE: Gary Lee, "Whistleblower Clears the Air," *Washington Post*, March 1, 1994, https://www.washingtonpost.com/archive/politics/1994/03/01/whistle-blower-clears-the-air/cc89bf64-180d-43f7-8373-9a6d410cef0d/. For a video from the National Whistleblower Center of the press conference after the trial, visit www.Marcus.ProjectFree.Me.

27. Dr. Phyllis Mullenix left her job at Harvard Medical School to establish the toxicology department at Forsyth Dental Center in Boston, the first toxicology department of any dental research institution in the world. After the director

encouraged her to study fluoride, she and her team were shocked when the research indicated that fluoride can cause both hyperactivity and hypoactivity in rats, depending on the stage of neural development during which the rats were exposed to fluoridated drinking water. SOURCE: Phyllis Mullenix, Pamela Denbesten, Ann Schunior, and William Kernan, "Neurotoxicity of Sodium Fluoride in Rats," *Neurotoxicology and Teratology* 17, no. 2 (March–April 1995): 169–77.

28. Phyllis Mullenix, "Fluoride and the Brain: An Interview with Dr. Phyllis Mullenix," interview by Paul Connett, Fluoride Action Network, October 18, 1997, available at http://fluoridealert.org/content/mullenix-interview/.

29. Despite previous claims from the U.S. Public Health Service (PHS) that fluoride is an essential mineral nutrient, researchers have been unable to identify any known side effects for consuming a diet deficient in fluoride, even with relation to dental health. As a result, "fluoride is no longer considered an essential factor for human growth and development." SOURCE: National Research Council (NRC), *Health Effects of Ingested Fluoride* (Washington, D.C.: National Academies Press, 1993). According to the Food and Drug Administration, fluoride is a drug "when used in the diagnosis, cure, mitigation, treatment, or prevention of disease in man or animal," For more information, see www.Drug.ProjectFree.Me.

30. The U.S. Deparment of Agriculture (USDA) and the Food and Drug Administration (FDA) are responsible for monitoring pesticide residue. Despite the establishment of a tolerance set for fluoride by the EPA, neither the FDA nor the USDA include fluoride-based pesticides on the list of pesticides they test for in their pesticide monitoring programs. In a 2014 report to Congress, the Government Accountability Office criticized the FDA for not disclosing in its annual report that inspectors do not

monitor for several common pesticides with established residue tolerances. SOURCE: Government Accountability Office, *FDA and USDA Should Strengthen Pesticide Residue Monitoring Programs and Further Disclose Monitoring Limitations*, GAO 15-38 (October 2014), https://www.gao.gov/assets/670/666408.pdf.

31. In response to a request from a pesticide manufacturer to exempt raisins from the residue tolerance for fluoride, EPA states, "Fluoride is naturally present in both food and water in varying amounts, and has been added to public water supplies to fight dental caries... Food contributes only small amounts of fluoride and monitoring the diet for fluoride intake is not very useful for current public health concerns." SOURCE: Environmental Protection Agency, *Notice of Filing a Pesticide Petition to Establish a Tolerance for a Certain Pesticide Chemical in or on Food*, Federal Register 66, No. 116 (June 15, 2001): 32618-21, available at www.EPA.ProjectFree.Me.

32. Researchers from Oregon State University measured the fluoride content of various foods made with mechanically deboned poultry. Pureed infant foods were highest in fluoride, up to 8.63 ppm, with a single serving containing up to 87 percent of the upper "safe" limit for fluoride for a six-month-old infant. Chicken sticks were the next highest, up to 6 ppm, with a single serving providing over half a milligram of fluoride. SOURCE: Noelle Fein and Florian Cerklewski, "Fluoride Content of Foods Made with Mechanically Separated Chicken," *Journal of Agricultural and Food Chemistry* 49, no. 9 (2001): 4284-86, available at www.Chicken.ProjectFree.Me.

33. Melissa Gallico, "How to Keep Your Dentist from Killing Your Labrador Retriever (and Other Pets)," Medium.com, June 2016, available at www.Raisins.ProjectFree.Me.

* To sign the petition, visit www.Petition.ProjectFree.Me

www.ingramcontent.com/pod-product-compliance
Lightning Source LLC
Chambersburg PA
CBHW080632030426
42336CB00018B/3167